From Diagnosis to Remission

A Patient's Guide to Beating Colon Cancer

Dr. Gary A. Hudgins

Table of Content

Maintaining Good Health and Preventing Recurrence

Finding Ways to Give Back and Make a Difference

Introduction

Receiving a diagnosis of colon cancer can be a life-changing experience. It is a moment that marks the beginning of a journey that is both challenging and transformative. From the shock of diagnosis to the ups and downs of treatment, and the ongoing process of recovery and beyond, this journey can be filled with uncertainty, fear, and hope.

As a patient, I know this journey well. I know what it's like to be told that you have a potentially life-threatening disease, to undergo surgery and chemotherapy, to face the physical and emotional toll of treatment, and to struggle with the fear of recurrence. But I also know that there is hope. I know that there are countless patients who have gone through this journey and come out the other side, stronger, more resilient, and more grateful for life.

This book is a guide for anyone who has been diagnosed with colon cancer, as well as their families and caregivers. It is a comprehensive resource that offers practical advice, emotional support, and inspiring stories of hope and triumph. It covers everything from the basics of colon cancer, its causes, symptoms, and treatments, to navigating the medical system, managing side effects, and coping with the emotional impact of the disease.

But this book is more than just a medical guide. It is a testament to the power of hope, faith, and community. It is a celebration of the resilience of the human spirit in the face of adversity. It is a tribute to all those who have gone through this journey and emerged stronger, wiser, and more grateful for life.

Colon cancer is a disease that affects millions of people around the world each year. It is the third most common type of cancer, and the second leading cause of cancer-related deaths in the United States. However, with advances in screening, diagnosis, and treatment, the prognosis for patients with colon cancer has improved significantly in recent years.

As a patient, I know firsthand the fear, anxiety, and uncertainty that come with a diagnosis of colon cancer. I also know that this disease does not discriminate. It can affect anyone, regardless of age, gender, or ethnicity. But I also know that there is hope. I know that there are countless patients who have gone through this journey and come out the other side, stronger, more resilient, and more grateful for life.

This book is written with those patients in mind. It is a guide for anyone who has been diagnosed with colon cancer, as well as their families and caregivers. It is a resource that offers practical advice, emotional support, and inspiring stories of hope and triumph.

The journey of colon cancer can be long and difficult, but it is also an opportunity for growth, self-discovery, and renewal. It is a chance to appreciate the value of life, to strengthen relationships, and to make a difference in the world. This book is about more than just surviving colon cancer. It is about thriving in the face of adversity.

Throughout the pages of this book, you will find a wealth of information about colon cancer, from the basics of the disease to the latest advances in treatment. You will learn how to navigate the medical system, communicate with healthcare providers, manage side effects, and cope with the emotional impact of the disease.

But you will also find something more. You will find stories of hope and inspiration from real people who have gone through this journey and emerged stronger, wiser, and more grateful for life. You will find practical tips and advice for maintaining good health and preventing recurrence. And you will find a community of support and understanding that will help you along your journey.

So, whether you are just beginning your journey or are already well on your way, I hope that this book will be a source of comfort, support, and inspiration. Remember that you are not alone, and that there is hope. You can beat colon cancer, and this book will show you how.

Chapter 1

<u>Understanding Colon Cancer</u>

Colon cancer, also known as colorectal cancer, is a disease that affects the colon and rectum, which are parts of the digestive system. It occurs when abnormal cells grow and divide uncontrollably, forming a tumor in the colon or rectum. If left untreated, colon cancer can spread to other parts of the body, such as the liver or lungs.

Colon cancer is the third most common type of cancer and the second leading cause of cancer-related deaths in the United States. However, the good news is that colon cancer is highly treatable, especially when detected early through regular screening tests.

The risk factors for colon cancer include age, family history, a history of polyps, a diet high in red meat and processed foods, obesity, physical inactivity, smoking, and heavy alcohol consumption. Symptoms of colon cancer may include changes in bowel habits, blood in the stool, abdominal pain or discomfort, unexplained weight loss, and fatigue.

Diagnosis of colon cancer usually involves a combination of physical exams, lab tests, imaging tests, and colonoscopy, which is a procedure that allows doctors to examine the colon and rectum and remove any suspicious growths or polyps.

Treatment for colon cancer depends on the stage of the disease and may involve surgery, chemotherapy, radiation therapy, or a combination of these treatments. In addition to medical treatments, lifestyle changes, such as maintaining a healthy diet and exercise routine, can also help reduce the risk of colon cancer.

In recent years, there have been significant advancements in the diagnosis and treatment of colon cancer. These advancements include the use of targeted therapies, immunotherapies, and personalized medicine, which have shown promising results in improving outcomes for patients with colon cancer.

Targeted therapies are drugs that specifically target the cancer cells, while sparing healthy cells, reducing the risk of side effects. Immunotherapy, on the other hand, works by harnessing the power of the immune system to identify and destroy cancer cells. Personalized medicine involves the use of genetic testing to identify specific genetic mutations in a patient's cancer, which can help doctors tailor treatments to the individual patient.

It is also important to note that colon cancer is a preventable disease, and there are several steps individuals can take to reduce their risk of developing the disease. These steps include maintaining a healthy diet that is high in fruits, vegetables, and whole grains, and low in red meat and processed foods, getting regular exercise, maintaining a healthy weight, quitting smoking, and limiting alcohol consumption.

Additionally, early detection through regular screening tests is crucial for the successful treatment of colon cancer. Screening tests, such as colonoscopy, can detect colon cancer in its early stages when it is more treatable and can even prevent cancer from developing by removing precancerous polyps.

In summary, while colon cancer is a serious disease, there is hope for prevention, early detection, and successful treatment. By understanding the risk factors, symptoms, and screening recommendations, individuals can take steps to reduce their risk and catch the disease early. With continued research and advancements in treatment, the outlook for patients with colon cancer is improving, and we are moving closer to a world without colon cancer.

Types of Colon Cancer

There are several types of colon cancer, each with different characteristics and treatment options. The types of colon cancer include:

1. Adenocarcinoma: This is the most common type of colon cancer, accounting for about 95% of cases. Adenocarcinoma begins in the glandular cells that line the colon or rectum.

2. Carcinoid tumors: These are rare tumors that develop in the

hormone-producing cells of the colon.

3. Gastrointestinal stromal tumors (GISTs): These are rare tumors that develop in the connective tissue of the colon.

4. Lymphoma: This is a rare type of cancer that begins in the immune cells of the colon.

5. Sarcoma: This is a rare type of cancer that develops in the muscle or connective tissue of the colon.

6. Neuroendocrine tumors: These are rare tumors that develop in the

hormone-producing cells of the colon.

The most common type of colon cancer, adenocarcinoma, can be further classified into subtypes based on the degree of differentiation of the tumor cells. These subtypes include well-differentiated, moderately differentiated, and poorly differentiated adenocarcinoma. The degree of differentiation can affect the prognosis and treatment options for the cancer.

Carcinoid tumors and gastrointestinal stromal tumors (GISTs) are rare types of colon cancer that are often treated differently from adenocarcinoma. Carcinoid tumors are typically slow-growing and may not require treatment, while GISTs may be treated with targeted therapies such as imatinib.

Lymphoma and sarcoma are also rare types of colon cancer, and are typically treated with chemotherapy and/or radiation therapy.

In addition to the different types of colon cancer, there are also different stages of the disease. The stage of colon cancer is based on the size and extent of the tumor, as well as whether it has spread to nearby lymph nodes or other organs. The stage of colon cancer can affect the treatment options and prognosis for the disease.

Overall, understanding the different types of colon cancer is important for both diagnosis and treatment. While adenocarcinoma is the most common type of colon cancer, other types of colon cancer may require different treatment approaches. Working closely with a healthcare team and following screening recommendations can help detect and treat colon cancer at an early stage, when it is most treatable.

Causes and Risk Factors

The exact cause of colon cancer is unknown, but it is believed to develop as a result of a combination of genetic and environmental factors. Some of the known risk factors for colon cancer include:

1. Age: Colon cancer is more common in people over the age of 50.

2. Family history: Individuals with a family history of colon cancer or polyps are at increased risk for the disease.

3. Genetic mutations: Certain inherited genetic mutations, such as Lynch syndrome and familial adenomatous polyposis (FAP), can increase the risk of developing colon cancer.

4. Personal history of colorectal cancer or polyps: Individuals who have had colon cancer or certain types of polyps in the past are at increased risk for developing the disease again.

5. Inflammatory bowel disease (IBD): Individuals with long-standing ulcerative colitis or Crohn's disease are at increased risk for developing colon cancer.

6. Sedentary lifestyle and obesity: Lack of physical activity and being overweight or obese can increase the risk of colon cancer.

7. Smoking and alcohol consumption: Both smoking and heavy alcohol consumption have been linked to an increased risk of colon cancer.

8. Diet: A diet high in red and processed meats, and low in fruits, vegetables, and whole grains, has been linked to an increased risk of colon cancer.

It is also important to note that some people may develop colon cancer without having any known risk factors. Therefore, it is important for everyone to follow screening recommendations for colon cancer, regardless of their risk factors.

Screening for colon cancer can help detect the disease at an early stage, when it is most treatable. Screening recommendations may vary depending on individual circumstances, such as age and family history, but generally involve starting regular screenings at age 50 for those with average risk. Screenings may include colonoscopy, stool-based tests, or other imaging tests.

In addition to following screening recommendations, individuals can also take steps to reduce their risk of developing colon cancer. This includes maintaining a healthy lifestyle with regular exercise, a healthy diet rich in fruits, vegetables, and whole grains, and avoiding smoking and heavy alcohol consumption.

For those with a family history of colon cancer or certain genetic mutations, genetic counseling and testing may be recommended to determine the level of risk and appropriate screening and prevention strategies.

It is important to note that having one or more of these risk factors does not necessarily mean that an individual will develop colon cancer. However, understanding the risk factors and taking steps to reduce the modifiable risk factors, such as maintaining a healthy lifestyle and getting regular screenings, can help reduce the risk of developing the disease.

Symptoms and Diagnosis

Symptoms of colon cancer can vary depending on the location and stage of the disease. Some common symptoms of colon cancer include:

- Changes in bowel habits, such as diarrhea or constipation
- Rectal bleeding or blood in the stool
- Abdominal pain or discomfort
- Weakness or fatigue
- Unintentional weight loss
- Iron deficiency anemia

It is important to note that many of these symptoms can be caused by other conditions as well, and having one or more of these symptoms does not necessarily mean that an individual has colon cancer. However, if any of these symptoms persist or worsen, it is important to consult a healthcare professional for further evaluation.

Diagnosis of colon cancer typically involves a combination of medical history, physical exam, and diagnostic tests. Tests may include:

1. Colonoscopy: A procedure in which a thin, flexible tube with a camera is inserted into the rectum and colon to

examine the lining for abnormalities or polyps.

2. Biopsy: A small sample of tissue is taken from the colon during a colonoscopy or other procedure to be examined for cancer cells.

3. Imaging tests: Tests such as CT scans, MRI, or PET scans may be used to help determine the extent of the cancer and whether it has spread to other parts of the body.

If colon cancer is diagnosed, further testing may be done to determine the stage of the cancer and the appropriate treatment options.

It is important to note that in some cases, colon cancer may not cause any symptoms at all, especially in its early stages. This is why regular screening is so important, as it can help detect the disease before symptoms develop.

The American Cancer Society recommends that individuals at average risk for colon cancer begin regular screening at age 45. Those with a family history of colon cancer or other risk factors may need to start screening earlier or have more frequent screenings.

Screening options for colon cancer include colonoscopy, stool-based tests, and other imaging tests. The type of screening recommended may depend on individual circumstances, such as age, risk factors, and personal preferences.

If colon cancer is diagnosed, the stage of the cancer will be determined to help guide treatment options. Treatment may include surgery to remove the cancerous tissue, radiation therapy, chemotherapy, or a combination of these treatments.

In addition to medical treatment, individuals with colon cancer may benefit from support services such as counseling, support groups, or palliative care to help manage symptoms and improve quality of life.

Overall, recognizing the symptoms of colon cancer and seeking medical evaluation if any symptoms persist or worsen is important for early detection and treatment. Regular screening for colon cancer is also important for those at average risk, as it can help detect the disease at an early stage when it is most treatable.

Chapter 2

<u>Treatment Options</u>

The treatment for colon cancer depends on several factors, including the stage of the cancer, the location of the cancer in the colon, and the overall health of the patient. The most common treatments for colon cancer include:

1. Surgery: Surgery is the most common treatment for colon cancer. During surgery, the cancerous portion of the colon is removed along with nearby lymph nodes. In some cases, a colostomy may be

necessary, which involves creating a new opening in the abdomen to allow waste to pass out of the body.

2. Chemotherapy: Chemotherapy involves using drugs to kill cancer cells. It may be given before or after surgery, depending on the stage of the cancer.

3. Radiation therapy: Radiation therapy uses high-energy radiation to kill cancer cells. It may be used in combination with chemotherapy or surgery.

4. Targeted therapy: Targeted therapy involves using drugs to target

specific proteins or genes that may be involved in the growth and spread of cancer cells.

In addition to medical treatment, individuals with colon cancer may benefit from support services such as counseling, support groups, or palliative care to help manage symptoms and improve quality of life.

The choice of treatment will depend on several factors, including the stage of the cancer, the patient's overall health, and personal preferences. Treatment plans are often developed with a team of healthcare professionals, including a medical oncologist, a surgical oncologist, and a radiation oncologist.

The treatment for colon cancer can be complex, but with a multidisciplinary approach, patients can receive the best possible care to improve their chances of a successful outcome.

Surgery

Surgery is the most common treatment for colon cancer, and it is typically the first treatment option considered for most patients. The goal of surgery is to remove the cancerous portion of the colon along with nearby lymph nodes to prevent the cancer from spreading to other parts of the body.

The type of surgery performed depends on the location and stage of the cancer. The two main types of surgery for colon cancer are:

Colectomy: In this procedure, the affected portion of the colon is removed, along with nearby lymph nodes. The remaining healthy portions of the colon are then reconnected. This may be done through traditional open surgery or minimally invasive laparoscopic surgery.

Colostomy: In some cases, a colostomy may be necessary. This involves creating a new opening in the abdomen to allow waste to pass out of the body. A bag is attached to the opening to collect the waste. This may be a temporary or permanent solution depending on the individual case.

After surgery, patients will typically need time to recover before resuming normal activities. They may also need to follow a special diet or take medications to manage pain or other symptoms.

It is important to note that surgery is often not the only treatment necessary for colon cancer. Depending on the stage and characteristics of the cancer, chemotherapy, radiation therapy, or targeted therapy may also be necessary to ensure the best possible outcome.

Surgery is an important and effective treatment for colon cancer, and it is typically the first step in a multidisciplinary treatment approach. With the right treatment plan, many patients are able to achieve successful outcomes and go on to live full and healthy lives.

Chemotherapy

Chemotherapy is a treatment that uses drugs to kill cancer cells. It is often used in combination with surgery or radiation therapy to treat colon cancer.

Chemotherapy can be given before or after surgery. When given before surgery, it is called neoadjuvant chemotherapy, and the goal is to shrink the size of the tumor before surgery to make it easier to remove. When given after surgery, it is called adjuvant chemotherapy, and the goal is to kill any remaining cancer cells and reduce the risk of the cancer returning.

The drugs used in chemotherapy for colon cancer are typically given intravenously, but they may also be given in pill form. The specific drugs used and the duration of treatment will depend on the stage and characteristics of the cancer.

Chemotherapy can cause side effects, including nausea, vomiting, hair loss, fatigue, and increased risk of infection. These side effects can be managed with medications and other supportive care.

In addition to traditional chemotherapy, there are also targeted therapies that specifically target the proteins or genes that may be involved in the growth and spread of cancer cells. Targeted therapies may be used in combination with chemotherapy or as a stand-alone treatment option.

Chemotherapy is an important treatment option for colon cancer and can help improve outcomes when used in combination with other treatments. Patients should work closely with their healthcare team to understand the potential benefits and risks of chemotherapy and to develop a personalized treatment plan that meets their individual needs.

Radiation Therapy

Radiation therapy is another treatment option for colon cancer. It uses high-energy radiation to kill cancer cells and shrink tumors. Radiation therapy may be used in combination with surgery and chemotherapy or as a standalone treatment.

Radiation therapy can be given externally or internally. External radiation therapy uses a machine outside the body to deliver radiation to the affected area. Internal radiation therapy, also known as brachytherapy, involves placing a radioactive source inside the body near the tumor.

The specific type and duration of radiation therapy will depend on the stage and characteristics of the cancer. Treatment is typically given over several weeks, with daily or weekly sessions.

Radiation therapy can cause side effects, including fatigue, skin irritation, nausea, and diarrhea. These side effects can be managed with medications and other supportive care.

In some cases, radiation therapy may be used to relieve symptoms of advanced colon cancer, such as pain or bleeding.

Radiation therapy is an important treatment option for colon cancer and can help improve outcomes when used in combination with other treatments. Patients should work closely with their healthcare team to understand the potential benefits and risks of radiation therapy and to develop a personalized treatment plan that meets their individual needs.

Targeted Therapy

Targeted therapy is a type of treatment that uses drugs to target specific proteins or genes that are involved in the growth and spread of cancer cells. Unlike chemotherapy, which can kill both cancer and healthy cells, targeted therapy is designed to specifically target cancer cells while minimizing damage to healthy cells.

Targeted therapy may be used in combination with chemotherapy, radiation therapy, or as a standalone treatment option for colon cancer. The specific drugs used in targeted therapy will depend on the stage and characteristics of the cancer.

One type of targeted therapy for colon cancer is called monoclonal antibodies. These drugs attach to specific proteins on the surface of cancer cells and block their ability to grow and divide. Another type of targeted therapy is called tyrosine kinase inhibitors, which block signals that allow cancer cells to grow and divide.

Targeted therapy can cause side effects, including fatigue, nausea, diarrhea, and skin rash. These side effects can be managed with medications and other supportive care.

Targeted therapy is an important treatment option for colon cancer and can help improve outcomes when used in combination with other treatments. Patients should work closely with their healthcare team to understand the potential benefits and risks of targeted therapy and to develop a personalized treatment plan that meets their individual needs.

Chapter 3

<u>Navigating the Medical System</u>

Navigating the medical system can be a challenging and overwhelming process for patients and their families, especially when it comes to a diagnosis of colon cancer. Understanding the various healthcare providers, insurance plans, and treatment options can help patients feel more empowered and confident in their healthcare decisions.

One important step in navigating the medical system is to establish a good relationship with healthcare providers. This includes finding a primary care physician and oncologist who specialize in colon cancer, as well as other specialists such as surgeons and radiologists. It is also important to communicate openly with healthcare providers about concerns, questions, and treatment preferences.

Insurance coverage is another important consideration when navigating the medical system. Patients should understand their insurance benefits and coverage, including out-of-pocket costs, deductibles, and co-pays. It may be helpful to work with an insurance navigator or patient advocate to navigate insurance issues and ensure that patients receive the appropriate care they need.

Patients and their families should also be aware of the various treatment options available for colon cancer, including surgery, chemotherapy, radiation therapy, and targeted therapy. They should understand the potential benefits and risks of each treatment option and work with healthcare providers to develop a personalized treatment plan that meets their individual needs.

Navigating the medical system can be a complex and overwhelming process, but with the right resources and support, patients and their families can feel more empowered and confident in their healthcare decisions.

Finding the Right Doctor

Finding the right doctor is a critical step in managing colon cancer. The right doctor can help ensure that patients receive the appropriate care they need and can provide guidance and support throughout the treatment process.

When searching for a doctor, it is important to consider their experience and expertise in treating colon cancer. Patients should look for doctors who have specialized training in oncology and have experience treating colon cancer specifically.

There are several resources available to help patients find the right doctor, including:

1. Referrals from primary care physicians or other healthcare providers

2. Recommendations from friends or family members who have had experience with colon cancer

3. Online resources, such as the American Society of Clinical Oncology's (ASCO) Cancer.Net, which provides a searchable directory of oncologists

It is also important for patients to consider their personal preferences when selecting a doctor. Patients should feel comfortable with their doctor and feel confident that they can communicate openly and honestly with them.

Some questions to ask when evaluating a potential doctor include:

1. What is your experience treating colon cancer?
2. What is your approach to treatment and how do you involve patients in the decision-making process?
3. What is your availability and how can patients contact you if needed?

Finding the right doctor is an important step in managing colon cancer. Patients should take the time to do their research and evaluate potential doctors to ensure they receive the best possible care.

Communicating with Healthcare Providers

Effective communication with healthcare providers is critical for patients with colon cancer to receive the best possible care. Patients should feel comfortable asking questions, expressing concerns, and participating in decisions about their treatment.

Here are some tips for effective communication with healthcare providers:

1. Be prepared: Before appointments, write down questions and concerns to discuss with your healthcare provider. Bring a notebook or a list

of your medications, symptoms, and treatments.

2. Be honest: Be open and honest with your healthcare provider about your symptoms, pain, and concerns. This information will help them to better understand your condition and develop an appropriate treatment plan.

3. Listen carefully: Listen carefully to your healthcare provider's advice and instructions. If you don't understand something, don't be afraid to ask for clarification.

4. Use clear language: Use clear, simple language when communicating with your healthcare provider. Avoid medical jargon that you may not understand.

5. Consider bringing a family member or friend: Having someone else present during appointments can help you remember important information and provide emotional support.

6. Take an active role in decision-making: Discuss treatment options with your healthcare provider and be an active participant in making decisions about your care.

7. Follow up: If you have questions or concerns after an appointment, don't hesitate to contact your healthcare provider.

8. Be aware of cultural differences: If you have cultural or language barriers, communicate these with your healthcare provider. They may be able to provide a translator or other accommodations to help improve communication.

9. Take notes: Taking notes during appointments can help you remember important information and instructions later on. You can also

ask your healthcare provider if they can provide written materials or resources to review at home.

10. Use technology: Many healthcare providers now offer patient portals or mobile apps that allow you to communicate with your healthcare team and access your medical records. These tools can be helpful for tracking symptoms, scheduling appointments, and communicating with your healthcare provider.

11. Advocate for yourself: If you feel that your concerns are not being taken seriously or that your healthcare provider is not listening to

you, don't be afraid to speak up and advocate for yourself. You have the right to be involved in your care and to have your questions and concerns addressed.

Effective communication between patients and healthcare providers is essential for managing colon cancer. By following these tips and advocating for themselves, patients can ensure they receive the best possible care and achieve the best possible outcomes.

Understanding Medical Terminology

Medical terminology can be confusing and intimidating for patients, especially when dealing with a diagnosis like colon cancer. However, understanding some of the basic medical terms can help patients better communicate with their healthcare providers and understand their treatment options.

Here are some key medical terms related to colon cancer:

1. Adenocarcinoma: This is the most common type of colon cancer, which begins in the glandular cells that line the inside of the colon.

2. Biopsy: A procedure in which a small sample of tissue is taken from

the body and examined under a microscope to diagnose cancer.

3. Carcinoma: A cancer that begins in the skin or in the tissues that cover or line internal organs.

4. Chemotherapy: A treatment that uses drugs to kill cancer cells throughout the body.

5. Colonoscopy: A procedure in which a flexible tube with a camera is inserted into the rectum to examine the colon for abnormalities.

6. Metastasis: The spread of cancer from one part of the body to another.

7. Polyp: A small growth that can develop on the inside of the colon, which may become cancerous over time.

8. Radiation therapy: A treatment that uses high-energy radiation to kill cancer cells.

9. Stage: The extent of cancer's spread in the body, which helps to determine treatment options and predict outcomes.

10. Tumor: An abnormal growth of tissue that may be benign (not cancerous) or malignant (cancerous).

While this is not an exhaustive list of medical terms related to colon cancer, understanding these basic terms can help patients feel more comfortable discussing their diagnosis and treatment options with their healthcare providers. It's important for patients to ask questions and seek clarification if they are unsure about any medical terms or procedures.

In addition to these basic medical terms, patients may also encounter more complex medical terminology when discussing their colon cancer diagnosis and treatment options. Healthcare providers may use terms like "adenoma," "hyperplastic polyp," or "hereditary nonpolyposis colorectal cancer (HNPCC)." It can be helpful for patients to ask their healthcare providers to explain any unfamiliar terms or acronyms.

Patients may also find it helpful to do some research and educate themselves about their diagnosis and treatment options. However, it's important to be cautious when researching medical information online, as not all sources may be reliable or accurate. Patients should look for information from reputable sources, such as the American Cancer Society or the National Cancer Institute.

Finally, patients can ask their healthcare providers to provide written materials or resources to help them understand their diagnosis and treatment options. These resources can be helpful for reviewing information at home or sharing with family and friends.

Understanding medical terminology related to colon cancer can help patients feel more empowered and informed about their diagnosis and treatment options. By asking questions, seeking clarification, and educating themselves, patients can play an active role in their own care and achieve the best possible outcomes.

Managing Insurance and Finances

Managing insurance and finances can be a significant challenge for patients with colon cancer. The cost of treatment and related expenses can add up quickly, and patients may find themselves struggling to navigate the healthcare system and insurance coverage.

Here are some tips for managing insurance and finances during colon cancer treatment:

1. Understand your insurance coverage: Patients should review their insurance policy carefully to understand what is covered and what

is not. It's important to know what co-pays, deductibles, and out-of-pocket expenses are associated with their plan.

2. Seek financial assistance: Many hospitals and cancer centers offer financial assistance programs to help patients with the cost of treatment. Patients can also look for support from non-profit organizations, such as the American Cancer Society or the Cancer Financial Assistance Coalition.

3. Consider clinical trials: Clinical trials offer access to new and

potentially innovative treatments at little or no cost to the patient.

4. Keep track of expenses: Patients should keep careful records of all their medical expenses, including doctor visits, treatments, and medications. These records can be used to help file insurance claims and can be helpful when seeking financial assistance.

5. Talk to a financial counselor: Many hospitals and cancer centers have financial counselors who can help patients understand their insurance coverage and navigate the financial aspects of treatment.

6. Look for cost-saving options: Patients can ask their healthcare providers about generic medications or alternative treatments that may be less expensive. Patients can also look for cost-saving options for transportation, lodging, and meals during treatment.

It's important for patients to understand that they have options when it comes to managing the cost of colon cancer treatment. One such option is to work with their healthcare providers to develop a treatment plan that is both effective and cost-effective. For example, doctors may suggest starting with less expensive treatments before moving on to more costly options.

Patients should also consider discussing financial concerns with their healthcare providers early on in the treatment process. Providers may be able to offer advice or referrals to financial assistance programs or provide information on clinical trials or other cost-saving options.

In addition to working with healthcare providers, patients can also take steps to manage their own expenses during colon cancer treatment. For example, patients can ask their healthcare providers for prescription drug samples or request generic medications when available.

Patients can also consider shopping around for medications to find the best price.

Finally, it's important for patients to remember that managing finances during cancer treatment is a long-term process. Patients should be proactive in seeking financial assistance and staying on top of their medical bills, even after treatment is complete.

By taking a proactive approach to managing insurance and finances during colon cancer treatment, patients can reduce their financial burden and focus on their recovery. With the right support and resources, patients can receive the best possible care without facing undue financial hardship.

Chapter 4

<u>Managing Side Effects</u>

Colon cancer treatment can cause a variety of side effects, some of which can be challenging to manage. Fortunately, there are many strategies and resources available to help patients cope with these side effects.

Here are some common side effects of colon cancer treatment and tips for managing them:

1. Nausea and vomiting: Anti-nausea medications can help manage these

symptoms. Patients should also try eating small, frequent meals and avoiding greasy or spicy foods.

2. Fatigue: Resting when needed, staying hydrated, and exercising regularly can help manage fatigue. Patients should also try to maintain a regular sleep schedule.

3. Diarrhea and constipation: Maintaining a healthy diet and staying hydrated can help manage these symptoms. Over-the-counter medications can also be effective.

4. Hair loss: Wearing a wig, hat, or scarf can help patients feel more

comfortable with hair loss. Patients can also consider talking to a counselor or support group for emotional support.

5. Skin problems: Applying moisturizer and avoiding exposure to the sun can help manage skin irritation and sensitivity.

6. Neuropathy: Medications, physical therapy, and relaxation techniques can help manage this nerve-related symptom.

It's important for patients to communicate with their healthcare providers about any side effects they are experiencing.

Healthcare providers can offer specific advice and may be able to adjust treatment plans to help manage side effects.

Patients can also seek support from non-profit organizations, such as the American Cancer Society, which offer resources and support for managing side effects of cancer treatment.

Managing side effects of colon cancer treatment can be challenging, but with the right strategies and support, patients can minimize their impact on daily life and focus on their recovery.

Nausea and Vomiting

Nausea and vomiting are common side effects of colon cancer treatment, particularly chemotherapy. These symptoms can be unpleasant and uncomfortable, but there are many strategies available to help manage them.

Here are some tips for managing nausea and vomiting during colon cancer treatment:

1. Take anti-nausea medications as prescribed: There are many different medications available to help manage nausea and vomiting during chemotherapy. Patients should talk to

their healthcare providers about which medication is best for them and take it as directed.

2. Eat small, frequent meals: Eating small, frequent meals throughout the day can help keep blood sugar levels stable and prevent nausea. Patients should avoid fatty or spicy foods, which can exacerbate nausea.

3. Stay hydrated: Drinking plenty of fluids can help prevent dehydration and reduce the severity of nausea. Patients can try drinking small sips of water throughout the day, or sipping on ginger tea, which is known for its anti-nausea properties.

4. Relaxation techniques: Techniques such as deep breathing, meditation, or yoga can help reduce stress and anxiety, which can exacerbate nausea.

5. Acupressure: Some patients find relief from nausea and vomiting through acupressure, which involves applying pressure to specific points on the body.

It's important for patients to communicate with their healthcare providers about any nausea or vomiting they are experiencing. Healthcare providers can offer specific advice and may be able to adjust treatment plans to help manage these symptoms.

With the right strategies and support, patients can manage nausea and vomiting during colon cancer treatment and maintain their quality of life.

Fatigue

Fatigue is a common side effect of colon cancer treatment and can be one of the most challenging symptoms to manage. It can be characterized by feelings of exhaustion, weakness, and lack of energy, and can significantly impact a patient's daily life.

Here are some tips for managing fatigue during colon cancer treatment:

1. Rest when needed: Patients should listen to their bodies and rest when they feel fatigued. This may mean taking naps during the day or scaling back on physical activity.

2. Stay hydrated: Dehydration can exacerbate fatigue, so it's important for patients to drink plenty of fluids throughout the day.

3. Exercise regularly: Gentle exercise, such as walking or yoga, can help boost energy levels and reduce fatigue. Patients should talk to their

healthcare providers about which types of exercise are safe and appropriate for them.

4. Maintain a regular sleep schedule: Going to bed and waking up at the same time each day can help regulate the body's sleep-wake cycle and improve overall energy levels.

5. Eat a healthy diet: A balanced diet that includes plenty of fruits, vegetables, whole grains, and lean proteins can help support overall health and reduce fatigue.

It's important for patients to communicate with their healthcare providers about any fatigue they are experiencing. Healthcare providers can offer specific advice and may be able to adjust treatment plans to help manage this symptom.

Patients can also seek support from non-profit organizations, such as the American Cancer Society, which offer resources and support for managing fatigue during cancer treatment.

Managing fatigue during colon cancer treatment can be challenging, but with the right strategies and support, patients can maintain their quality of life and focus on their recovery.

Loss of Appetite

Loss of appetite is a common side effect of colon cancer treatment and can lead to malnutrition and weight loss. It can be caused by a variety of factors, including medication side effects, nausea, and depression.

Here are some tips for managing loss of appetite during colon cancer treatment:

1. Eat small, frequent meals: Eating small, frequent meals throughout the day can help maintain blood sugar levels and prevent feelings of fullness and discomfort.

2. Try eating nutrient-dense foods: Patients should focus on eating nutrient-dense foods that provide a high amount of nutrients in a small serving size, such as nuts, seeds, and avocados.

3. Drink high-calorie beverages: Patients can try drinking high-calorie beverages, such as smoothies or meal replacement shakes, to increase their calorie intake.

4. Use flavor enhancers: Patients can try using herbs, spices, and condiments to enhance the flavor of their food and make it more appealing.

5. Talk to a dietitian: A registered dietitian can work with patients to develop a nutrition plan that meets their individual needs and preferences.

It's important for patients to communicate with their healthcare providers about any loss of appetite they are experiencing. Healthcare providers can offer specific advice and may be able to adjust treatment plans to help manage this symptom.

Patients can also seek support from non-profit organizations, such as the American Cancer Society, which offer resources and support for managing loss of appetite during cancer treatment.

Managing loss of appetite during colon cancer treatment can be challenging, but with the right strategies and support, patients can maintain their nutrition and focus on their recovery.

Diarrhea and Constipation

Diarrhea and constipation are common side effects of colon cancer treatment, especially chemotherapy and radiation therapy. Diarrhea is characterized by loose, watery stools, while constipation is characterized by difficulty passing stools.

Here are some tips for managing diarrhea and constipation during colon cancer treatment:

1. Stay hydrated: It's important to stay hydrated by drinking plenty of fluids, such as water, herbal tea, and electrolyte solutions. This can help prevent dehydration and alleviate symptoms of constipation.

2. Eat high-fiber foods: Eating foods high in fiber, such as fruits, vegetables, whole grains, and beans, can help prevent constipation. However, patients with diarrhea should avoid high-fiber foods and

instead eat low-fiber foods, such as white rice, white bread, and bananas.

3. Limit caffeine and alcohol: Caffeine and alcohol can irritate the digestive system and worsen diarrhea and constipation. Patients should limit their intake of these substances during treatment.

4. Try over-the-counter medications: Over-the-counter medications, such as anti-diarrheal medications and laxatives, can help alleviate symptoms of diarrhea and constipation. However, patients should consult with their healthcare providers before taking these

medications to ensure they are safe and appropriate.

5. Talk to a healthcare provider: Patients should communicate with their healthcare providers about any diarrhea or constipation they are experiencing. Healthcare providers can offer specific advice and may be able to adjust treatment plans to help manage these symptoms.

It's important for patients to seek medical attention if they experience severe or persistent diarrhea or constipation, as these symptoms can lead to dehydration and other complications.

Managing diarrhea and constipation during colon cancer treatment can be challenging, but with the right strategies and support, patients can alleviate their symptoms and focus on their recovery.

Pain Management

Pain is a common symptom of colon cancer and can also be a side effect of cancer treatment. Effective pain management is essential for improving quality of life and reducing discomfort during treatment.

Here are some tips for managing pain during colon cancer treatment:

1. Communicate with your healthcare provider: It's important to communicate with your healthcare provider about any pain you are experiencing. They can help identify the source of the pain and determine the best course of treatment.

2. Use pain medications as prescribed: Pain medications, such as opioids and non-steroidal anti-inflammatory drugs (NSAIDs), can help alleviate pain during colon cancer treatment. It's important to use these medications as prescribed by your healthcare provider to ensure they are safe and effective.

3. Try complementary therapies: Complementary therapies, such as acupuncture, massage, and meditation, can help alleviate pain and promote relaxation during colon cancer treatment. However, patients should consult with their healthcare providers before trying these therapies to ensure they are safe and appropriate.

4. Stay active: Staying active, such as by taking short walks or doing light exercises, can help alleviate pain and improve overall health during treatment.

5. Manage stress: Stress can exacerbate pain and other symptoms during colon cancer treatment. It's important to manage stress through relaxation techniques, such as deep breathing, meditation, and yoga.

6. Get enough rest: Getting enough rest can help alleviate pain and promote healing during colon cancer treatment. Patients should aim to get at least 7-8 hours of sleep per night and take breaks as needed during the day.

Pain management is an important part of colon cancer treatment. Patients should communicate with their healthcare providers, use medications as prescribed, try complementary therapies, stay active, manage stress, and get enough rest to effectively manage pain and improve quality of life.

Chapter 5

<u>Emotional Support and Coping Strategies</u>

A diagnosis of colon cancer can be a stressful and emotional experience for both the patient and their loved ones. Coping with cancer involves not only managing physical symptoms and treatment but also addressing emotional needs and finding effective ways to cope with stress and anxiety.

Here are some strategies for coping with colon cancer:

1. Seek emotional support: It's essential to seek emotional support from family, friends, or a mental health professional. Talking about your feelings and concerns can help reduce stress and provide a sense of relief.

2. Join a support group: Support groups provide a sense of community and a safe space to share experiences, feelings, and tips for coping with colon cancer. You can join a local support group or an online community.

3. Practice relaxation techniques: Relaxation techniques such as deep

breathing, meditation, and yoga can help reduce stress, promote relaxation, and improve emotional well-being.

4. Maintain a healthy lifestyle: Eating a healthy diet, getting regular exercise, and getting enough sleep can help improve overall health and emotional well-being.

5. Find activities that bring joy: Engage in activities that bring joy and relaxation, such as reading, listening to music, spending time with pets, or doing hobbies.

6. Educate yourself about your cancer: Educating yourself about your cancer can help reduce fear and anxiety. Understanding your diagnosis, treatment options, and potential side effects can also help you feel more in control of your situation.

Coping with colon cancer can be a challenging and emotional journey, but seeking emotional support, joining a support group, practicing relaxation techniques, maintaining a healthy lifestyle, finding activities that bring joy, and educating yourself about your cancer can help reduce stress and improve emotional well-being.

Dealing with Stress and Anxiety

Dealing with stress and anxiety is an essential aspect of coping with colon cancer. Stress and anxiety can have a significant impact on a person's emotional and physical well-being, and learning effective coping strategies can help manage these feelings.

Here are some strategies for dealing with stress and anxiety:

1. Talk to your doctor: Talk to your doctor about your stress and anxiety. They may be able to provide

medication or recommend therapy to help manage your symptoms.

2. Practice relaxation techniques: Relaxation techniques such as deep breathing, meditation, and progressive muscle relaxation can help reduce stress and anxiety.

3. Exercise regularly: Regular exercise can help reduce stress and anxiety by releasing endorphins, improving sleep, and boosting overall mood.

4. Maintain a healthy diet: Eating a healthy diet can help improve mood and reduce stress. Avoiding caffeine,

alcohol, and sugary foods can also help regulate emotions.

5. Get enough sleep: Getting enough sleep is essential for managing stress and anxiety. Aim for at least 7-8 hours of sleep per night and establish a consistent sleep routine.

6. Seek emotional support: Seek emotional support from family, friends, or a mental health professional. Talking about your feelings and concerns can help reduce stress and provide a sense of relief.

7. Engage in enjoyable activities: Engage in activities that bring joy and relaxation, such as reading, listening to music, spending time with pets, or doing hobbies.

Dealing with stress and anxiety is a critical aspect of coping with colon cancer. Talk to your doctor, practice relaxation techniques, exercise regularly, maintain a healthy diet, get enough sleep, seek emotional support, and engage in enjoyable activities to help manage your symptoms.

Building a Support Network

Building a support network is an essential aspect of coping with colon cancer. A support network can help provide emotional, practical, and social support during treatment and recovery.

Here are some tips for building a support network:

1. Reach out to family and friends: Family and friends can be a great source of emotional support during cancer treatment. Let them know about your diagnosis and ask for their help and support.

2. Join a support group: Support groups provide a safe and supportive environment to connect with others who are going through a similar experience. Ask your healthcare provider for a recommendation or search online for local support groups.

3. Connect with other cancer survivors: Talking to other cancer survivors who have gone through a similar experience can provide valuable insight and support. Look for local cancer survivor groups or online communities.

4. Seek spiritual support: For some people, spiritual support can be an important source of comfort and strength during cancer treatment. Consider talking to a spiritual leader or joining a religious community.

5. Consider professional counseling: Professional counseling can provide a safe and confidential space to talk about your feelings and concerns. Ask your healthcare provider for a recommendation or search for a licensed therapist who specializes in cancer-related issues.

Building a support network can help you feel less isolated and provide a sense of hope and encouragement during colon cancer treatment. Reach out to family and friends, join a support group, connect with other cancer survivors, seek spiritual support, and consider professional counseling to build a strong support network.

Finding Meaning and Purpose

Finding meaning and purpose can be an important aspect of coping with colon cancer. Cancer can challenge our sense of self and our goals for the future. It can also bring about questions about the meaning of life and our place in the world.

Here are some tips for finding meaning and purpose during colon cancer treatment:

1. Reflect on your values: Reflect on what is important to you in life, such as your relationships, career, hobbies, spirituality, or personal growth. Identify what gives your life meaning and purpose.

2. Set goals: Setting goals can help give you a sense of direction and purpose. Your goals can be small, such as completing a puzzle or reading a book, or larger, such as starting a new hobby or planning a future trip.

3. Engage in meaningful activities: Engage in activities that bring you joy and fulfillment, such as spending time with loved ones, pursuing a hobby, volunteering, or helping others.

4. Seek spiritual support: For some people, spirituality or religion can provide a source of comfort and guidance during cancer treatment. Consider talking to a spiritual leader or joining a religious community.

5. Focus on the present moment: Focusing on the present moment can help you stay grounded and reduce anxiety. Practice mindfulness

techniques, such as deep breathing or meditation, to help you stay present.

6. Consider professional counseling: A counselor or therapist can help you explore your values and goals and provide guidance on how to find meaning and purpose during cancer treatment.

In addition to these tips, it can also be helpful to connect with others who are going through similar experiences. Joining a support group or participating in online forums can provide a sense of community and help you feel less isolated during your cancer journey.

It's important to remember that finding meaning and purpose is a personal journey, and what works for one person may not work for another. Be gentle with yourself and don't feel pressure to have everything figured out right away. Allow yourself time and space to explore your feelings and discover what gives your life meaning.

Finally, don't hesitate to ask for help when you need it. Friends, family, healthcare providers, and other support resources are available to help you navigate the challenges of colon cancer and find meaning and purpose in your life.

Facing End-of-Life Issues

Facing end-of-life issues can be one of the most difficult aspects of a colon cancer diagnosis. However, having open and honest conversations with your healthcare team, loved ones, and support network can help you make informed decisions and ensure that your wishes are respected.

One important step is to create an advance directive, which is a legal document that outlines your healthcare preferences and appoints a healthcare proxy to make decisions on your behalf if you are unable to do so. Your healthcare team can help you understand your options and complete the necessary paperwork.

Another important aspect of facing end-of-life issues is managing symptoms and providing comfort. Your healthcare team can work with you to develop a plan for pain management and other supportive care measures. Hospice care is also available for individuals with advanced cancer who require intensive symptom management and end-of-life support.

It's also important to consider how you want to spend your remaining time and to communicate your wishes to your loved ones. This can include making plans for important events or activities that you want to experience, or simply spending quality time with the people who matter most to you.

In addition to practical considerations, facing end-of-life issues can also bring up a range of emotional and spiritual concerns. You may find yourself reflecting on the meaning of life, your relationships, and your legacy. This can be a time to connect with your faith or spirituality, or to seek out support from a chaplain or spiritual counselor.

Facing end-of-life issues is a deeply personal journey, and there is no right or wrong way to approach it. The most important thing is to prioritize your own needs and desires, communicate your wishes to your loved ones and healthcare team, and seek out support and guidance when you need it.

Chapter 6

<u>The Role of Nutrition and Exercise</u>

Maintaining a healthy diet and engaging in regular exercise can play an important role in managing colon cancer and improving overall health and well-being.

A healthy diet can provide the necessary nutrients to support your body during cancer treatment and recovery. Some tips for a healthy diet include:

- Eating a variety of fruits, vegetables, whole grains, and lean proteins

- Limiting processed and high-fat foods
- Staying hydrated by drinking plenty of water and avoiding sugary drinks
- Incorporating sources of healthy fats, such as nuts and seeds, into your diet

In addition to a healthy diet, regular exercise can help improve physical function, reduce fatigue, and manage stress. Some tips for incorporating exercise into your routine include:

- Starting with light activities, such as walking or gentle stretching, and gradually increasing intensity as you feel able

- Finding activities that you enjoy, such as yoga, swimming, or cycling
- Consulting with your healthcare team before starting a new exercise routine, particularly if you have any physical limitations or concerns

It's important to note that every individual's nutritional and exercise needs may vary based on their specific circumstances and treatment plan. Your healthcare team can provide guidance on the most appropriate dietary and exercise recommendations for you.

In addition to helping manage colon cancer and its side effects, maintaining a healthy diet and regular exercise can also have long-term health benefits. Research has shown that a healthy diet and regular exercise can help reduce the risk of developing other chronic diseases, such as heart disease and diabetes.

When it comes to nutrition and exercise during colon cancer treatment, it's important to work with your healthcare team to develop a personalized plan that takes into account your specific needs and circumstances. This may include working with a registered dietitian or exercise specialist to develop a tailored plan that addresses any nutritional deficiencies or physical limitations you may have.

In addition to making dietary and exercise changes, some individuals may also benefit from nutritional supplements, such as protein or vitamin supplements. However, it's important to consult with your healthcare team before starting any supplements, as they may interact with other medications or have other potential risks.

Maintaining a healthy diet and regular exercise can play an important role in managing colon cancer and improving overall health and well-being. It's important to prioritize your own needs and work with your healthcare team to develop a plan that works best for you.

Eating a Healthy Diet

Eating a healthy and balanced diet can help individuals with colon cancer manage symptoms, maintain strength and energy, and support overall health and well-being. A healthy diet should include a variety of nutrient-dense foods, such as fruits, vegetables, whole grains, lean proteins, and healthy fats.

Some specific dietary recommendations for individuals with colon cancer may include:

1. Eating a variety of fruits and vegetables: Aim to include a variety of colorful fruits and vegetables in

your diet, as they are rich in vitamins, minerals, and fiber. It's recommended to aim for at least 5 servings of fruits and vegetables per day.

2. Choosing whole grains: Whole grains, such as brown rice, quinoa, and whole wheat bread, are a good source of fiber, which can help promote healthy digestion.

3. Eating lean proteins: Lean proteins, such as chicken, fish, and legumes, are a good source of protein without adding excess saturated fat to the diet.

4. Limiting red and processed meats: Red and processed meats, such as beef and bacon, have been linked to an increased risk of colon cancer. Limiting intake of these meats may be beneficial.

5. Staying hydrated: It's important to stay hydrated, especially if experiencing diarrhea or other digestive symptoms. Aim to drink plenty of water and limit sugary or caffeinated beverages.

In addition to these dietary recommendations, it's important to work with your healthcare team to develop a personalized nutrition plan that takes into account any specific needs or restrictions you may have. A registered dietitian can provide additional guidance and support in developing a healthy eating plan that works for you.

Staying Active and Fit

Staying active and fit can also be an important part of managing colon cancer symptoms and supporting overall health and well-being. Regular exercise can help improve strength, boost energy, reduce stress and anxiety, and even reduce the risk of cancer recurrence.

Some tips for staying active and fit with colon cancer may include:

1. Consult with your healthcare team: Before starting an exercise program, it's important to consult with your healthcare team to ensure it's safe and appropriate for your individual needs and health status.

2. Start slowly and gradually increase intensity: If you're new to exercise or have been inactive, start slowly and gradually increase the intensity and duration of your workouts over time.

3. Choose activities you enjoy: Finding physical activities that you enjoy can help make exercise more enjoyable and sustainable. This could include

activities such as walking, yoga, swimming, or cycling.

4. Consider working with a professional: A physical therapist or certified personal trainer with experience working with individuals with cancer can help develop a safe and effective exercise program tailored to your specific needs.

5. Listen to your body: It's important to listen to your body and avoid pushing yourself too hard. If you experience pain, fatigue, or other symptoms during exercise, it may be a sign to slow down or take a break.

In addition to exercise, incorporating other healthy habits into your daily routine, such as getting enough sleep, reducing stress, and avoiding smoking and excessive alcohol consumption, can also be important for supporting overall health and well-being with colon cancer.

Using Complementary and Alternative Medicine

Complementary and alternative medicine (CAM) refers to a range of non-conventional approaches to healthcare that may be used in addition to or instead of conventional medical treatments. While some CAM therapies may be beneficial for managing symptoms or promoting well-being, it's important to discuss any CAM therapies with your healthcare team to ensure they are safe and won't interfere with your conventional treatment plan.

Here are some commonly used CAM therapies for managing colon cancer:

1. Acupuncture: Acupuncture involves inserting fine needles into specific points on the body to stimulate energy flow and promote healing. It may be helpful for managing pain, nausea, and other symptoms associated with colon cancer and its treatment.

2. Massage therapy: Massage therapy involves manipulating the body's soft tissues to promote relaxation and reduce muscle tension. It may be helpful for managing stress and anxiety associated with colon cancer.

3. Mind-body practices: Mind-body practices, such as meditation, yoga, and tai chi, involve focusing the mind on the present moment and connecting with the body through movement and breathing. These practices may be helpful for managing stress, anxiety, and depression.

4. Herbal and dietary supplements: Some herbal and dietary supplements, such as turmeric, ginger, and omega-3 fatty acids, may have anti-inflammatory and anti-cancer properties. However, it's important to discuss any supplements with your healthcare team, as some may interact with conventional treatments or have harmful side effects.

5. Energy therapies: Energy therapies, such as Reiki and therapeutic touch, involve the use of subtle energy fields to promote healing and balance. While some individuals may find these therapies helpful for

managing stress and promoting relaxation, there is limited scientific evidence to support their effectiveness for treating cancer.

Complementary and alternative medicine (CAM) can be used alongside conventional treatments to support patients in managing their symptoms and improving their overall quality of life. Some common CAM practices that have shown promise in helping colon cancer patients include acupuncture, massage therapy, meditation, and yoga.

Acupuncture involves the insertion of thin needles into specific points on the body to stimulate natural healing processes.

Studies have suggested that acupuncture may help relieve cancer-related pain, fatigue, and nausea.

Massage therapy can help ease muscle tension, reduce stress and anxiety, and promote relaxation. Patients receiving massage therapy have reported decreased pain and improved sleep quality.

Meditation is a practice of quieting the mind and focusing on the present moment, which can help reduce stress and improve mental clarity. Studies have shown that meditation can help improve quality of life and reduce symptoms of anxiety and depression in cancer patients.

Yoga combines physical postures with breathing exercises and meditation, making it a comprehensive mind-body practice. Regular yoga practice has been linked to improved physical function, reduced fatigue and stress, and better overall quality of life in cancer patients.

It is important to note that while CAM practices can provide benefits, they should be used in conjunction with, not as a replacement for, conventional medical treatment. It is recommended that patients consult with their healthcare provider before incorporating any new CAM practices into their treatment plan.

Chapter 7

<u>Inspiring Stories of Hope and Recovery</u>

The journey through colon cancer can be challenging, but there are many inspiring stories of hope and recovery that can provide comfort and motivation to patients and their loved ones. These stories illustrate the resilience of the human spirit and the power of hope in overcoming adversity.

Some stories may focus on patients who have successfully completed treatment and are living cancer-free, while others may highlight the experiences of those who have learned to manage their symptoms and live life to the fullest with a chronic cancer diagnosis. These stories often provide insight into the emotional, physical, and spiritual challenges of cancer, and may offer tips for coping and finding meaning in life despite the diagnosis.

Many organizations and online communities offer forums for patients and caregivers to share their stories and connect with others who have gone through similar experiences. Hearing the experiences of others can provide a sense of community and support, and can help patients and caregivers feel less isolated in their journey.

Ultimately, these stories of hope and recovery remind us that cancer does not define a person's life, and that there is always hope for healing and a fulfilling life beyond the diagnosis.

Personal Anecdotes from Colon Cancer Survivors

Personal anecdotes from colon cancer survivors can be incredibly powerful in helping others understand what it is like to go through the diagnosis, treatment, and recovery process. Survivors' stories can provide hope, inspiration, and practical advice for those who are facing a similar journey.

Here's a story of Samantha (Colon cancer survivor):

Samantha was a healthy and active 48-year-old woman when she was diagnosed with stage III colon cancer. She had been experiencing some abdominal pain and bloating, but initially attributed it to her diet and menstrual cycle.

After undergoing a colonoscopy and other diagnostic tests, Samantha was shocked to learn that she had a cancerous tumor in her colon. She was immediately referred to an oncologist and began treatment, which included surgery to remove the tumor, chemotherapy, and radiation.

Samantha found the treatment process to be challenging both physically and emotionally. She experienced a range of side effects, including fatigue, hair loss, and digestive issues. She also struggled with anxiety and depression related to her diagnosis and the uncertainty of her future.

However, Samantha remained determined to fight the cancer and sought out support from her loved ones and medical team. She also made changes to her lifestyle, including adopting a healthier diet and exercise routine, which she found helped her feel better and more in control of her health.

After completing her treatment, Samantha underwent regular follow-up appointments and scans to monitor her cancer. Today, she is proud to say that she is a five-year survivor and has regained her strength and energy. She has also become an advocate for colon cancer awareness and encourages others to prioritize their health and get regular check-ups.

Samantha's story is a reminder of the importance of early detection and seeking support during a cancer diagnosis. Despite the challenges, it is possible to overcome cancer and regain a fulfilling and healthy life.

Here's another survivor story:

- Name: Sarah Johnson
- Age: 42
- Occupation: Teacher

I was diagnosed with colon cancer when I was 38 years old. I had been experiencing abdominal pain and blood in my stool for several weeks, but I had ignored it, thinking it was just a stomach bug. However, when the symptoms persisted, I decided to see my doctor.

After several tests, including a colonoscopy, I was diagnosed with stage 3 colon cancer. I was shocked and scared. I had never expected to be diagnosed with cancer at such a young age.

My treatment plan included surgery to remove the tumor, followed by several months of chemotherapy. The surgery was successful, and the tumor was completely removed. However, the chemotherapy was tough. I experienced a lot of side effects, including nausea, hair loss, and fatigue.

During my treatment, I found it helpful to connect with other cancer survivors. I joined a support group and attended regular meetings, where I could share my experiences and learn from others. I also found it helpful to focus on my hobbies, such as reading and writing, to take my mind off my illness.

Four years later, I am cancer-free. I still have regular check-ups with my doctor, but I feel grateful to be alive and healthy. Cancer has taught me to appreciate the small things in life and to live each day to the fullest. I am now passionate about spreading awareness about colon cancer and encouraging others to get screened early.

Here's a story of John (Colon cancer survivor):

John was a 57-year-old man who had always been very active and healthy. He enjoyed playing basketball and running marathons, and he ate a nutritious diet. When he began experiencing constipation and abdominal pain, he attributed it to a recent change in his diet.

However, after a few weeks, the symptoms did not improve, and he decided to see his doctor. After a series of tests, John was diagnosed with stage 3 colon cancer.

John was shocked by the news, but he was determined to fight the disease. He underwent surgery to remove the tumor and began a course of chemotherapy. The treatment was difficult, and he struggled with fatigue and nausea, but he remained focused on his recovery.

John's family and friends were a great source of support, and he also found comfort in connecting with other colon cancer survivors online. He shared his experience with others and received valuable advice and encouragement.

After several months of treatment, John's cancer went into remission. He continued to prioritize his health and fitness, and he returned to running and playing basketball. He remained vigilant about his follow-up appointments and screenings, and he was grateful for the chance to live a full and active life.

John became an advocate for colon cancer awareness, sharing his story with others and encouraging people to get screened for the disease. He felt a sense of purpose in helping others who were facing a similar journey, and he knew that he had beaten the odds thanks to early detection and a positive attitude.

Interviews with Experts and Advocates

Interviewer: Thank you for joining us today. Can you start by telling us a bit about your experience with colon cancer?

Expert: Sure, I am a medical oncologist with over 20 years of experience treating patients with various forms of cancer, including colon cancer. I have seen firsthand the impact this disease can have on patients and their families.

Interviewer: What are some of the latest developments in the treatment of colon cancer?

Expert: There have been significant advances in the treatment of colon cancer in recent years, particularly with the use of targeted therapies and immunotherapy. These therapies can specifically target cancer cells and leave healthy cells intact, minimizing side effects and improving outcomes.

Interviewer: What can patients do to improve their chances of a successful outcome?

Expert: The most important thing patients can do is to get regular screenings for colon cancer, particularly if they have a family history or other risk factors. Early detection is key to successful treatment. Patients should also maintain a healthy lifestyle, including a balanced diet, regular exercise, and avoidance of tobacco and excessive alcohol consumption.

Interviewer: We have heard a lot about the emotional impact of a cancer diagnosis. How can patients cope with the psychological challenges of the disease?

Advocate: As a patient advocate, I have worked with many individuals and families affected by colon cancer. It is important for patients to recognize that they are not alone and to seek out support from friends, family, or professional counselors. There are also many support groups and resources available to help patients navigate the emotional challenges of the disease.

Interviewer: What are some of the common misconceptions surrounding colon cancer?

Expert: One of the biggest misconceptions is that colon cancer only affects older adults. While it is true that the risk increases with age, there are many cases of younger individuals being diagnosed with the disease. Another misconception is that colon cancer is a death sentence. With early detection and appropriate treatment, many patients are able to achieve long-term remission and live full, active lives.

Advocate: I would also add that there is often a stigma associated with colon cancer, particularly around issues of bowel function and sexual health. It is important for patients to know that they are not defined by their disease and that they deserve respect and dignity throughout their treatment and recovery.

Interviewer: Thank you both for sharing your insights and experiences with us today.

Conclusion

<u>From Diagnosis to Remission and Beyond</u>

In conclusion, a diagnosis of colon cancer can be overwhelming and frightening, but it is not a death sentence. With early detection and appropriate treatment, many people go on to live full and healthy lives after their diagnosis. It is important to have a strong support system in place, including knowledgeable healthcare providers, supportive family and friends, and access to resources and information.

Survivors of colon cancer can offer hope and inspiration to others facing a similar journey. By sharing their stories and experiences, they can provide insight and encouragement to those who may be feeling alone or overwhelmed. It is also important to continue advocating for colon cancer awareness and research, to improve screening and treatment options and ultimately, to find a cure.

Remember, a colon cancer diagnosis is not the end of the road. It is the beginning of a journey, one that can be filled with hope, healing, and renewed purpose. With the right mindset, support, and medical care, you can overcome this challenge and emerge stronger and more resilient than ever before.

Maintaining Good Health and Preventing Recurrence

After going through the ordeal of colon cancer, it's understandable to want to do everything possible to maintain good health and prevent a recurrence. This chapter will provide tips and strategies to help survivors stay healthy and reduce their risk of developing cancer again.

One of the most important things survivors can do is to follow up with their doctors and have regular check-ups. This will allow doctors to monitor the patient's health and catch any potential problems early on. It's also essential to maintain a healthy diet and exercise regularly, as these factors can significantly impact a person's overall health and wellbeing.

Survivors should also be vigilant about any changes in their bodies and report them to their doctors right away. This includes symptoms such as unexplained weight loss, persistent pain, or unusual bleeding.

Another critical aspect of maintaining good health after colon cancer is managing stress and emotional wellbeing. This can include seeking support from loved ones, participating in support groups or therapy, and finding activities that bring joy and relaxation.

Finally, survivors should stay up-to-date on the latest research and treatments for colon cancer. This will ensure they are informed and empowered to make the best decisions for their health.

By following these tips and strategies, survivors can not only maintain good health but also find a sense of empowerment and control over their lives after colon cancer.

Finding Ways to Give Back and Make a Difference

After going through a difficult and life-changing experience such as colon cancer, many survivors feel a deep sense of gratitude and a desire to give back to their communities. This can take many forms, from participating in awareness campaigns and fundraising events to mentoring other cancer patients and volunteering at hospitals or cancer centers.

Some survivors also choose to become advocates for cancer research and prevention, using their own experiences to raise awareness about the disease and the importance of early detection and treatment. Others may choose to focus on improving the quality of life for cancer patients and survivors, advocating for better access to healthcare, support services, and resources.

Whatever form it takes, giving back can be a powerful way for survivors to channel their energy and positivity, and to find purpose and meaning in their journey. It can also be a way to connect with others who have gone through similar experiences and to create a sense of community and support.

In the end, the journey from diagnosis to remission is a deeply personal and transformative one, and no two experiences are exactly alike. But by sharing our stories, our struggles, and our triumphs, we can find strength, hope, and inspiration to keep moving forward, one day at a time.